OSTEOPOROSIS DIET COOK BOOK FOR SENIORS

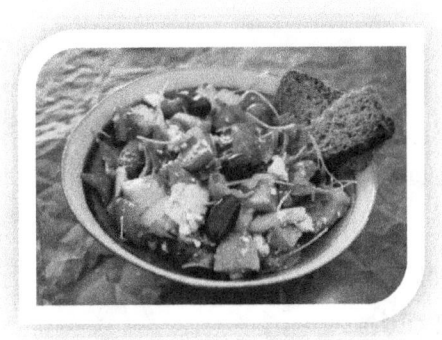

Nutrition Guide and Healthy Bone Rich - Calcium Recipes to Naturally Combat Osteoporosis

DR. ANA JONES

TABLE OF CONTENT

CHAPTER 3: _____ 35

CONCLUSION _____ 79

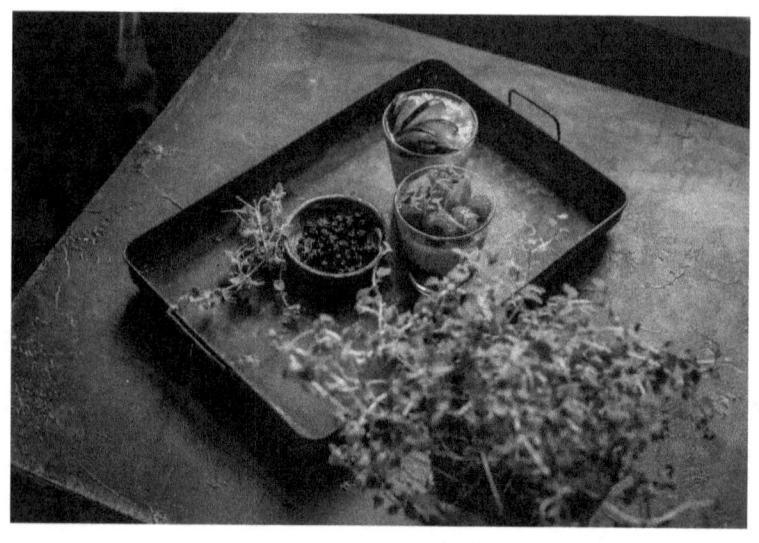

To the seniors bravely facing the challenges of osteoporosis,

In the quiet corridors of your strength, where resilience meets vulnerability, I see your courage shining like a beacon in the night. Each day, you navigate the labyrinth of pain and uncertainty with a grace that inspires awe. Your journey, marked by the silent struggles of osteoporosis, does not go unnoticed. Today, I dedicate these words to you, warriors of the spirit, whose battles are fought not with swords but with unwavering determination.

Osteoporosis, a thief in the night, may have stolen your ease of movement, but it will never lay claim to your indomitable spirit. In the depths of your bones, where fractures threaten to shatter dreams, I implore you to hold onto hope as fiercely as you hold onto life itself. For within the heart of adversity lies the seed of resilience, waiting to bloom into a garden of triumph.

Though the road may be fraught with obstacles, remember that you do not walk alone.

Each step you take is buoyed by the unwavering support of those who stand beside you, their love a steadfast anchor in the tempest of uncertainty. Lean on them when the burden feels too heavy, for together, you are an unstoppable force, capable of weathering any storm.

As the sun sets on another day, casting shadows that dance like memories across the canvas of your life, dare to believe in the promise of tomorrow. For in the darkest moments, when despair threatens to eclipse the light, it is hope that illuminates the path forward, guiding you towards a future filled with possibility.

So, dear seniors, as you navigate the labyrinth of osteoporosis, know that you are cherished, valued, and deeply admired. Your resilience is a testament to the power of the human spirit, a reminder that even in the face of adversity, there is always hope. May you find solace in the knowledge that within you burns a flame that can never be extinguished, lighting the way towards a brighter tomorrow.

INTRODUCTION

Welcome to a culinary journey that transcends mere recipes; welcome to a celebration of vitality, resilience, and the sheer joy of living well. As a seasoned nutritionist, I've dedicated decades to understanding the intricate dance between food and health, and I'm thrilled to present to you the culmination of my expertise: "Nourishing Bones, Savoring Life: "Osteoporosis Diet Cookbook for Seniors."

Within these pages, you'll discover more than just a collection of delectable dishes. You'll find a roadmap to fortifying your bones, enriching your life, and embracing each day with renewed vigor. Osteoporosis may pose its challenges, but armed with the right knowledge and nourishment,

we can defy its limitations and savor life to its fullest.

This cookbook isn't just about what to eat; it's about empowering you to reclaim control over your health and well-being. With carefully crafted recipes that prioritize calcium-rich ingredients, bone-strengthening nutrients, and flavors that delight the senses, every meal becomes an opportunity to nurture your body and indulge your palate.

But this journey isn't just about sustenance; it's about community, connection, and the joy of sharing a meal with loved ones. Whether you're dining solo or hosting a gathering of cherished friends, each recipe is a testament to the profound impact that food has on our lives – not just in terms of nourishment, but in fostering bonds, creating memories, and enriching our shared human experience.

So, let this cookbook be your trusted companion on the path to optimal bone health and vibrant living. Let it inspire you to embrace the power of nutrition, to savor each bite with gratitude, and to approach every day with the unwavering belief that a well-nourished body is capable of remarkable feats.

Together, let's embark on a journey of culinary discovery, where every meal is a testament to the resilience of the human spirit and the boundless possibilities that await when we prioritize our health.

"Osteoporosis Diet Cookbook for Seniors" isn't just a cookbook – it's a manifesto for living your best life, one delicious meal at a time.

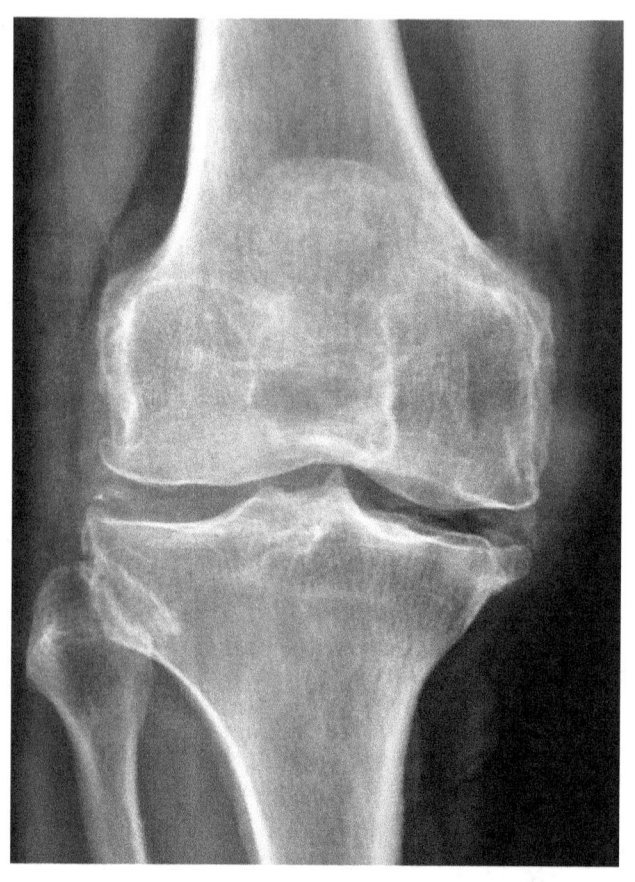

CHAPTER 1:

Understanding Osteoporosis

Called the "silent disease," osteoporosis is a prevalent bone-related disorder that is frequently misdiagnosed. Bones become weaker and thinner as a result of it, which increases their vulnerability to breaks and fractures. We will examine the different forms, causes, symptoms, and preventive methods of osteoporosis in this in-depth investigation, equipping you with the information to safeguard your own and your loved ones' bone health.

Types of osteoporosis

1. Primary Osteoporosis: This kind is more frequently linked to hormone fluctuations and age. There are two fundamental categories of primary osteoporosis: I. Osteoporosis following menopause: It mainly affects women after menopause and is caused by a decrease in estrogen, which is essential for preserving bone density.

II. Osteoporosis Associated with Age: This kind, which affects both men and women, is connected to aging naturally and the progressive loss of bone density over time.

2. Secondary Osteoporosis: This kind is brought on by drugs or underlying medical disorders that affect bone density.

Secondary osteoporosis can result from conditions like long-term steroid use, malabsorption disorders, and hyperparathyroidism.

Symptoms of osteoporosis

Osteoporosis frequently advances silently, showing no signs at all, until a fracture happens. Wrist, hip, and spinal fractures are the most frequent fractures linked to osteoporosis. Nonetheless, osteoporosis can present with a number of mild symptoms, such as:

1. Back Pain: This type of pain is chronic and is frequently brought on by fractures or the collapse of weaker vertebrae

2. Decrease of Height: Osteoporosis can cause a progressive decrease of height over time.

3. Sloped Posture: Also called "dowager's hump," this is caused by the curvature of the spine as a result of fractures.

4. Bone Fractures: Bone fractures can happen more frequently and with less force, particularly in the hip, wrist, or spine.

It's important to keep in mind that osteoporosis can go years without showing any symptoms, so getting tested for bone density as soon as possible is key.

Causes and symptoms of osteoporosis

It is essential to comprehend the underlying causes of osteoporosis for both management and prevention. The following are the main causes of osteoporosis development:

1. Aging: Our bones naturally lose density as we become older, making fractures more likely.

2. Hormonal Changes: Hormonal changes, especially the decrease in estrogen in postmenopausal women, are a major contributing factor to osteoporosis. A drop in testosterone levels in men may potentially be a factor in bone loss.

3. **Family History:** Having osteoporosis in one's family can raise one's risk.

4. **Nutritional Decisions:** Vitamin D insufficiency, inadequate calcium intake, and poor nutrition can all damage bones.

5. **Lifestyle Factors:** Sedentary behavior, smoking, drinking too much alcohol, and not getting enough exercise can all make bone loss worse.

6. **Medical illnesses:** Rheumatoid arthritis, gastrointestinal diseases, and hyperparathyroidism are a few medical illnesses that might cause secondary osteoporosis.

7. **Medication:** Corticosteroids, anticonvulsants, and some cancer treatments can all cause bone weakness over time.

Preventive measures for osteoporosis

Fortunately, there are a number of Lifestyle modifications and preventative actions that can lower the risk of osteoporosis:

1. **A Well-Balanced Diet:** To maintain strong bones, make sure your diet is high in calcium and vitamin D. Good sources include dairy products, leafy greens, and fortified meals.

2. **Frequent Exercise:** Weight-bearing activities that increase and maintain bone density include running, walking, and strength training.

3. **Lifestyle Decisions:** Limit alcohol intake and give up smoking, as both can exacerbate bone loss.

4. **Bone Density Testing:** Osteoporosis can be detected early with regular bone density scans, allowing for prompt intervention.

5. **Medication:** To control osteoporosis, doctors may occasionally advise using medication. These ought to be utilized with modifications to one's way of life.

6. **Fall Prevention:** Take precautions to lessen the chance of falling, such as installing handrails, making sure areas are well-lit, and clearing out any trip hazards from your home.

7. **Hormone Replacement Therapy:** In order to preserve bone density, postmenopausal women may want to think about hormone replacement therapy.

Understanding the different types, causes, symptoms, and preventive actions of osteoporosis is essential to managing this silent but serious danger to bone health.

You may fortify your bones, lower your risk of fractures, and live an active and independent retirement by leading a bone-healthy lifestyle and seeking early diagnosis and treatment when necessary. Recall that maintaining healthy bones is an investment in your general wellbeing.

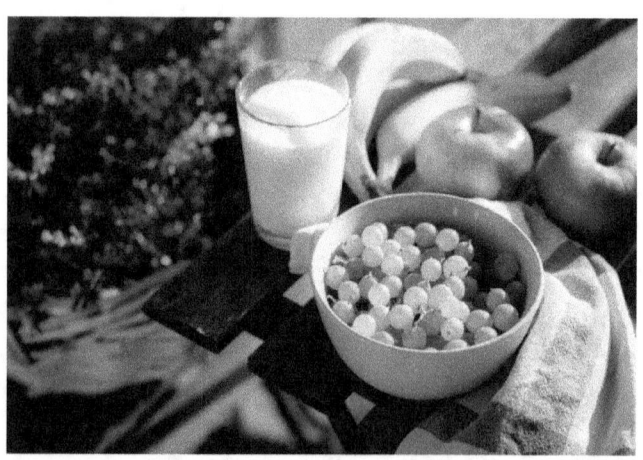

CHAPTER 2:

Benefit of following osteoporosis Diet for seniors

A senior's osteoporosis diet can provide a number of fundamental advantages that are critical for controlling and averting this condition. The main benefits are as follows:

Enhanced Bone Health: An osteoporosis diet emphasizes calcium as well as other vital elements that are critical for healthy bones, such as magnesium, vitamin K, and vitamin D. By slowing down bone loss, strengthening bones, and lowering the risk of fractures, consuming these nutrients eventually increases bone density.

Decreased Fracture Risk: Fractures are less common in strong bones. Seniors who follow a well-balanced diet and maintain optimal bone health can greatly reduce their chance of suffering from crippling fractures, which are particularly common in cases of osteoporosis.

Improved Muscle Function: A diet high in protein, especially from lean sources, promotes the health of your muscles. Robust muscles enhance general movement and assist elderly individuals in maintaining equilibrium, lowering the possibility of fractures from falls.

Improved Joint Health: Foods high in nutrients, such fruits and vegetables, have anti-inflammatory and antioxidant properties that can help treat joint pain and discomfort, which is frequently linked to osteoporosis.

Maintained Independence: Seniors who have strong bones and muscles are able to keep their independence and carry on with their everyday activities without the need for help. Higher living quality and more self-sufficiency result from this.

Enhanced Nutrient Absorption: Foods high in vitamin C and other nutrients that facilitate improved nutrient absorption are frequently included in an osteoporosis diet. This makes it easier for the body to absorb vital nutrients that strengthen bones.

Heart Health: A diet low in sodium and high in healthy fats, for example, is one of the many elements that promotes heart health in people with osteoporosis.

Better bone health and a lower risk of heart-related problems are two advantages that seniors can experience.

Weight management: Seniors can maintain a healthy weight by eating a balanced diet. Being underweight can raise the risk of fractures, while being overweight can place unneeded strain on the bones and joints. A constant, healthy weight is supported by an osteoporosis diet. Decrease in Dependency on.

Medication: A healthy diet may be able to lessen the requirement for osteoporosis drugs. This improves general health and well-being while also reducing the possibility of negative side effects.

Reduced Osteoporosis Progression: Seniors can reduce the rate at which osteoporosis develops by adopting an osteoporosis diet. This implies that they will be able to better regulate and manage the signs and consequences of osteoporosis.

Greater General Nutrition: Eating foods high in nutrients is encouraged by an osteoporosis diet,

which can increase general nutrition and general health. It assists elderly people in obtaining the vital vitamins and minerals required for optimum health.

Lower chance of Falls: Foods strong in protein and calcium, which promote muscle strength and balance, can help seniors retain their stability and lower their chance of falling, which is a significant cause of hip fractures in the elderly.

An osteoporosis diet for the elderly provides a comprehensive strategy for controlling and averting the illness. It not only helps with bone health but also with general health, self-sufficiency, and a higher standard of living. Seniors who focus important nutrients in their diet can greatly improve their physical health and lower their risk of issues associated to osteoporosis.

Osteoporosis foods to eat, limit and avoid

For general well-being, achieving and preserving good bone and joint health is critical, and managing osteoporosis makes this even more so. A well-planned diet might be an effective management strategy for this illness.

We'll look at foods that support strong bones and joints in this guide, including those to eat, avoid, and limit.

Foods to eat:

Nuts and Seeds: Rich sources of calcium, magnesium, and other minerals that are essential for strong bones include almonds, chia seeds, and sesame seeds.

Lean Proteins: To keep your muscles and bones strong, eat lean protein sources such beans, tofu, and chicken.

Whole Grains: Whole grains include vital nutrients including magnesium, which is important for bone health. Examples of these are brown rice and whole wheat bread.

Fruits: Vitamin C, found in fruits like oranges and berries, promotes the synthesis of collagen, which is essential for the health of bones and joints.

Dairy Products: Milk, yogurt, and cheese are examples of dairy products that are high in calcium, which is an essential component of bones. To limit your intake of saturated fat, choose low-fat or non-fat varieties.

Leafy Greens: Vitamin K, which promotes bone mineralization, and calcium are found in abundance in vegetables including kale, broccoli, and collard greens.

Fatty Fish: Rich in vitamin D and omega-3 fatty acids, which promote bone health, salmon, mackerel, and sardines are good sources of these nutrients.

Foods fortified: A lot of foods, such orange juice and fortified cereals, have extra calcium and vitamin D. These could be beneficial supplements to your diet.

Low-Fat Dairy Alternatives: Fortified almond milk, soy milk, or other alternatives enhanced with calcium and vitamin D are your best bets if you're lactose intolerant or prefer non-dairy options.

Foods to limit:

Sugary drinks and sodas: These frequently include phosphoric acid, which can obstruct the absorption of calcium. Make healthier beverage selections, such as herbal teas or water.

Alcohol: Drinking too much alcohol can weaken bones and raise the possibility of fractures. If you decide to drink, make sure it's moderate.

Red Meat: Lean cuts of meat are a good source of protein, but only in moderation. Consuming too much red meat can cause the body to become acidic, which may have an impact on bone health.

Salt: Diets high in sodium can cause the urine to lose calcium, which is bad for the health of the bones. Limit the amount of packaged and processed meals you eat to cut down on salt.

Caffeine: Consuming too much caffeine may cause the body to lose calcium. Reduce the amount of tea, coffee, and caffeinated soda you consume.

Foods to avoid:

Overindulgence in Sweets: Consuming too much sugar can cause inflammation and impair the body's capacity to absorb calcium.

Highly Acidic Foods: Meals that make the body's environment more acidic, including a lot of meat and some cereals, may be a factor in the weakening of bones.

Overly Salty Snacks: Consuming a lot of salty snacks, such as potato chips and pretzels, can increase sodium intake, which can cause calcium loss.

Highly Processed meals: Processed meals are frequently heavy in sugar, salt, and harmful fats, all of which can be detrimental to one's health, particularly the health of one's bones and joints.

Trans Fats: Often included in fried and processed meals, trans fats have the potential to lower bone density and cause inflammation.

For the health of your bones and joints, leading a healthy lifestyle is just as important as what you eat. Walk or do resistance training or other weight-bearing exercises to maintain muscle strength and promote bone formation. Enough vitamin D, obtained via sunshine exposure and supplements when needed, is also essential since it facilitates the body's effective absorption of calcium.

You can effectively manage osteoporosis and create a greater quality of life by adopting a holistic approach to bone and joint health and making mindful dietary choices. Recall that achieving stronger bones and better joints requires a balanced diet.

Complications of osteoporosis when the right diet isn't adopted

Osteoporosis can result in a number of grave consequences if the proper diet and management techniques are not used.

These issues have the potential to seriously affect a person's general health and quality of life.

The following are a few of the most typical side effects of poorly managed or untreated osteoporosis:

Kyphosis (Dowager's Hump): Kyphosis, also known as dowager's hump, is a condition where the spine curves forward as a result of several vertebral fractures. This alteration in posture can lead to respiratory problems and back pain in addition to physical appearance.

Hospitalization: Hospitalization and surgery are frequently necessary for fractures, especially hip fractures. For anyone, especially seniors, hospital stays can be emotionally and physically taxing.

Bone fractures are the main and most noticeable consequence of osteoporosis. Fractures are far more common in weaker bones, especially those of the hip, spine, and wrist. These fractures can cause discomfort, incapacity, and loss of independence. They can arise from even little falls or routine activity.

Chronic Back discomfort: Osteoporotic fractures, particularly those involving the vertebrae, can result in persistent back discomfort. A person's quality of life can be greatly diminished by this persistent pain, which can also make daily tasks challenging.

Reduced movement: Chronic pain and fractures can both cause a reduction in movement. This reduction in exercise can lead to balance issues and muscle weakness, which raises the risk of fractures and falls.

Surgical consequences: There are a number of risks and consequences associated with surgical methods for fracture repair, including the possibility of infection, blood clots, and problems connected to anesthesia.

Loss of Independence: Osteoporosis can cause a person to lose their independence due to discomfort, fractures, and restricted movement. Seniors may need help with everyday tasks, which can be upsetting emotionally.

Psychological Effects: Depression, worry, and a lowered sense of wellbeing are just a few of the severe psychological effects that osteoporosis-related issues can cause.

These emotional difficulties are exacerbated by loss of independence, changing body image, and chronic pain.

Reduced Quality of Life: Every one of the aforementioned issues leads to a lower standard of living. It could be difficult for people to exercise, participate in social events, or pursue past passions and hobbies.

Increased Healthcare Costs: Treating osteoporosis-related consequences, such as fractures, operations, and hospital stays, can result in high healthcare expenses, which can be expensive for both individuals and healthcare systems.

Risk of Further Fractures: After suffering an osteoporotic fracture, a person is more susceptible to further fractures. This is referred to as the "fracture cascade" and adds to the financial and health burden.

It's crucial to remember that osteoporosis is frequently avoidable and controllable with dietary adjustments, weight-bearing activity, and the right medical care. People can considerably lower their risk of problems and preserve their general health and bone health by receiving early detection and prompt treatment.

As such, it is imperative that those who are at risk of osteoporosis take preventive action.

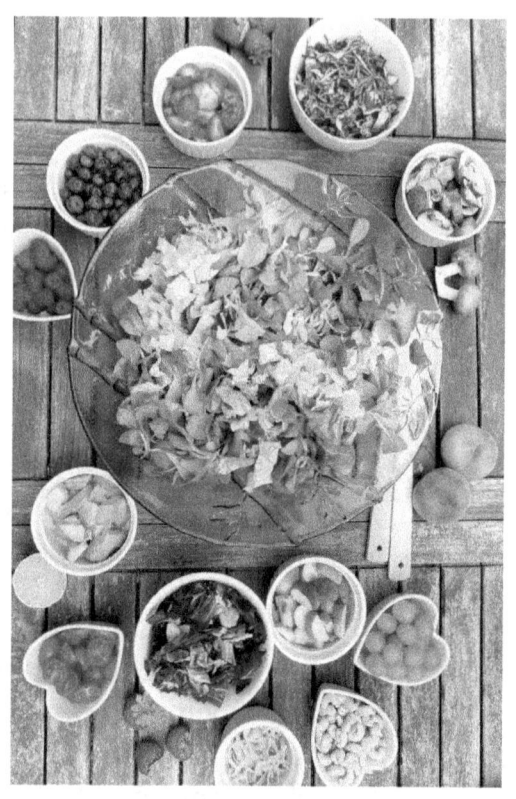

7 DAY MEAL PLAN

DAY 1:

BREAKFAST: **Banana and Almond Butter Smoothie**

(Page 35)

LUNCH: **Spinach and Salmon Salad**

(Page 48)

DINNER: **Turkey and Vegetable Stir-Fry**

(Page 55)

DAY 2:

BREAKFAST: **Blueberry and Almond Oatmeal**
(Page 38)

LUNCH: **Salmon and Vegetable Foil Pack**

(Page 46)

DINNER: **Chicken and Vegetable Skewers**

(Page 57)

DAY 3:

BREAKFAST: **Banana and Almond Butter Smoothie**

(Page 35)

LUNCH: **Sweet Potato and Kale Salad**

(Page 44)

DINNER: **Tofu and Vegetable Stir-Fry**

(Page 59)

DAY 4:

BREAKFAST: **Creamy Greek Yogurt Parfait**

(Page 39)

LUNCH: **Quinoa and Beakfast Bowl**

(Page 37)

DINNER: **Baked Lemon Herb Tilapia**

(Page 62)

DAY 5:

BREAKFAST: **Spinach and Feta Omelette**

(Page 40)

LUNCH: **Grilled Chicken and Asparagus**

(Page 51)

DINNER: **Quinoa and Vegetable Stuffed Bell Peppers**

(Page 63)

DAY 6:

BREAKFAST: **Avocado and Tomato Toast**

(Page 34)

LUNCH: **Broccoli and Chickpea Stir-Fry**

(Page 53)

DINNER: **Vegetable and Quinoa Soup**

(Page 61)

DAY 7:

BREAKFAST: **Cottage Cheese and Berries Bowl**
(Page 36)

LUNCH: **Tuna and White Bean Salad**

(Page 52)

DINNER: **Stuffed Acorn Squash**

(Page 56)

CHAPTER 3

BREAKFAST RECIPES:

1. Overnight Chia Seed Pudding

Ingredients:

- ❖ 3 tablespoons chia seeds
- ❖ 1 cup unsweetened almond milk
- ❖ 1/4 teaspoon vanilla extract
- ❖ 1/4 cup fresh berries
- ❖ 1 tablespoon chopped walnuts

Preparation:

1. In a jar, combine chia seeds, almond milk, and vanilla extract. Stir well.
2. Refrigerate the mixture for at least four hours or overnight.
3. Top with fresh berries and chopped walnuts before serving.

Serving: 1 serving

Nutritional Value: Calories: 220, Protein: 6g, Calcium: 350mg, Fiber: 10g

Cooking Time: 5 minutes (plus overnight refrigeration)

2. Avocado and Tomato Toast

Ingredients:

- ❖ 1 slice whole-grain bread
- ❖ 1/2 ripe avocado, mashed
- ❖ 1 small tomato, sliced
- ❖ Salt and pepper to taste

Preparation:

1. Toast the whole-grain bread.
2. Spread the mashed avocado on the toast.
3. Season with salt and pepper and serve with sliced tomatoes.

Serving: 1 serving

Nutritional Value:

Calories: 230

Protein: 5g

Calcium: 40mg

Fiber: 6g

Cooking Time: 5 minutes

3. Banana and Almond Butter Smoothie

Ingredients:

- ❖ 1 ripe banana
- ❖ 1 tablespoon almond butter
- ❖ 1 cup unsweetened almond milk
- ❖ 1/2 teaspoon cinnamon
- ❖ 1 teaspoon honey (optional)

Preparation:

1. Blend all of the ingredients in a blender until smooth.
2. Add honey (if desired) for extra sweetness.

Serving: 1 serving

Nutritional Value:

Calories: 280

Protein: 5g

Calcium: 200mg

Cooking Time: 5 minutes

4. Cottage Cheese and Berries Bowl

Ingredients:

- ❖ 1/2 cup low-fat cottage cheese
- ❖ 1/4 cup mixed berries (blueberries, strawberries, raspberries)
- ❖ 1 tablespoon chopped pecans
- ❖ 1/2 teaspoon honey (optional)

Preparation:

1. In a bowl, layer the cottage cheese and mixed berries.
2. Top with chopped pecans and drizzle with honey (if desired).

Serving: 1 serving

Nutritional Value:

Calories: 250,

Protein: 16g,

Calcium: 200mg

Cooking Time: 5 minutes

5. Quinoa Breakfast Bowl

Ingredients:

- ❖ 1/2 cup cooked quinoa
- ❖ 1/4 cup sliced peaches
- ❖ 1 tablespoon pumpkin seeds
- ❖ 1 teaspoon honey (optional)

Preparation:

1. In a bowl, place the cooked quinoa.
2. Top with sliced peaches and pumpkin seeds.
3. Drizzle with honey (if desired).

Serving: 1 serving

Nutritional Value: Calories: 280

Protein: 7g

Calcium: 40mg

Fiber: 4g

Cooking Time: 15 minutes (for quinoa preparation)

6. Blueberry and Almond Oatmeal

Ingredients:

- ❖ 1/2 cup old-fashioned oats
- ❖ 1 cup unsweetened almond milk
- ❖ 1/4 cup fresh blueberries
- ❖ 1 tablespoon sliced almonds
- ❖ 1/2 teaspoon honey (optional)

Preparation:

1. Cook oats with almond milk according to package instructions.
2. Top with fresh blueberries, sliced almonds, and a drizzle of honey (if desired).

Serving: 1 serving

Nutritional Value:

Calories: 280

Protein: 8g

Calcium: 200mg

Fiber: 6g

Cooking Time: 10 minutes

Ingredients:

- ❖ 1 cup plain Greek yogurt
- ❖ 1/4 cup sliced strawberries
- ❖ 1 tablespoon chopped almonds
- ❖ 1 teaspoon honey (optional)
- ❖ 1/2 teaspoon chia seeds

Preparation:

1. In a bowl, layer the Greek yogurt, strawberries, and almonds.
2. Drizzle honey (if desired) and sprinkle chia seeds on top and Serve immediately.

Serving: 1 serving

Nutritional Value:

Calories: 260

Protein: 18g

Calcium: 250mg

Fiber: 4g

Cooking Time: 5 minutes

Ingredients:

- ❖ 2 large eggs
- ❖ 1/4 cup fresh spinach, chopped
- ❖ 2 tablespoons crumbled feta cheese
- ❖ Salt and pepper to taste
- ❖ 1 teaspoon olive oil

Preparation:

1. In a mixing dish, whisk together the eggs and season with salt and pepper.
2. In a nonstick skillet, heat the olive oil over a moderate heat.
3. Add the spinach and Cook for about two minutes or until the spinach has wilted.
4. Pour the beaten eggs over the spinach and sprinkle feta cheese on top.
5. Cook until the omelette is set, then fold it in half and serve.

Serving: 1 serving

Nutritional Value: Calories: 270, Protein: 18g, Calcium: 140mg

Cooking Time: 10 minute

9. Almond and Berry Quinoa Breakfast Bowl

Ingredients:

- ❖ 1/2 cup cooked quinoa
- ❖ 1/4 cup mixed berries (strawberries, blackberries, blueberries)
- ❖ 2 tablespoons sliced almonds
- ❖ 1/2 teaspoon honey (optional)

Preparation:

1. In a bowl, place the cooked quinoa.
2. Top with mixed berries and sliced almonds.
3. Drizzle with honey (if desired).

Serving: 1 serving

Nutritional Value:

Calories: 290

Protein: 8g

Calcium: 60mg

Fiber: 6g

Cooking Time: 15 minutes (for quinoa preparation)

10. Sweet Potato and Spinach Breakfast Hash

Ingredients:

- ❖ 1 small sweet potato, diced
- ❖ 1 cup fresh spinach
- ❖ 1/4 cup diced red bell pepper
- ❖ 2 large eggs
- ❖ Salt and pepper to taste
- ❖ 1 teaspoon olive oil

Preparation:

1. In a pan, heat the olive oil over moderate heat.
2. Add diced sweet potato and cook until tender and slightly crispy, about 10 minutes.
3. Add in the red bell pepper and cook for two more minutes.
4. Add the fresh spinach, stir, and cook until it wilts.
5. Create two small wells in the hash and crack eggs into them.
6. Cook the eggs covered until they reach your desired liking.
7. Season with salt and pepper before serving.
   Serving: 2 servings

Nutritional Value (per serving):

Calories: 280

Protein: 11g

Calcium: 80mg

Cooking Time: 20 minutes

These simple and quick breakfast recipes are ideal for seniors with osteoporosis since they are heart- and diabetes-healthy and offer vital minerals for strong bones. They are full of vitamins and minerals that support healthy bones and general well-being, and they taste great and are easy to prepare.

1. Sweet Potato and Kale Salad

Ingredients:

- ❖ 1 cup roasted sweet potato cubes
- ❖ 2 cups chopped kale
- ❖ 1/4 cup dried cranberries
- ❖ 1/4 cup chopped pecans
- ❖ 1 tablespoon balsamic vinaigrette
- ❖ Salt and pepper to taste

Preparation:

1. In a bowl, combine roasted sweet potato, chopped kale, dried cranberries, and pecans.
2. Season with salt and pepper and drizzle with balsamic vinaigrette.

Serving: 1 serving

Nutritional Value: Calories: 310, Protein: 5g, Calcium: 80mg

Cooking Time: 30 minutes (for sweet potato roasting)

2. Egg and Vegetable Wrap

Ingredients:

- ❖ 2 large eggs, 1 whole-grain tortilla
- ❖ 1/4 cup diced bell peppers
- ❖ 1/4 cup diced onions
- ❖ 1/4 cup diced tomatoes
- ❖ 1/4 cup chopped spinach
- ❖ 1/4 cup low-fat cheese (optional)
- ❖ Salt and pepper to taste

Preparation:

1. In a mixing dish, whisk together the eggs and season with salt and pepper.
2. In a pan, sauté bell peppers, onions, and tomatoes until soft.
3. Add the beaten eggs and cook until set.
4. Lay the egg mixture on the tortilla, top with chopped spinach and cheese (if desired), and wrap.

Serving: 1 serving

Nutritional Value: Calories: 330, Protein: 17g, Calcium: 150mg

Cooking Time: 15 minutes

3. Salmon and Vegetable Foil Pack

Ingredients:

- ❖ 4 oz salmon fillet
- ❖ 1/2 cup broccoli florets
- ❖ 1/2 cup carrot slices
- ❖ 1/4 cup red onion slices
- ❖ 1/2 tablespoon olive oil
- ❖ 1/2 teaspoon lemon zest
- ❖ Salt and pepper to taste

Preparation:

1. Preheat the oven to 375°F (190°C).
2. Place salmon, broccoli, carrots, and red onions on a large piece of aluminum foil.
3. Drizzle with olive oil and lemon zest, and season with salt and pepper.
4. Seal the foil into a packet and bake for 20-25 minutes, until the salmon is cooked through.

Serving: 1 serving

Cooking Time: 25 minutes

Nutritional Value: Calories: 320, Protein: 25g, Calcium: 150mg

4. Mediterranean Hummus Wrap

Ingredients:

- ❖ 1 whole-grain tortilla
- ❖ 2 tablespoons hummus
- ❖ 2 slices roasted red pepper
- ❖ 1/4 cup cucumber slices
- ❖ 1/4 cup mixed greens
- ❖ 1/4 cup crumbled feta cheese (optional)

Preparation:

1. Spread hummus on the whole-grain tortilla.
2. Layer with roasted red pepper, cucumber slices, mixed greens, and crumbled feta cheese (if desired).
3. Roll up the tortilla into a wrap.

Serving: 1 serving

Nutritional Value: Calories: 280, Protein: 8g, Calcium: 100mg

Cooking Time: 10 minutes

5. Spinach and Salmon Salad

Ingredients:

- ❖ 3 oz cooked salmon
- ❖ 2 cups fresh spinach
- ❖ 1/4 cup cherry tomatoes
- ❖ 1/4 cup cucumber slices
- ❖ 1 tablespoon olive oil and lemon juice
- ❖ Salt and pepper to taste

Preparation:

1. Flake the cooked salmon and set it aside.
2. In a large bowl, combine fresh spinach, cherry tomatoes, and cucumber slices.
3. Season with salt and pepper after drizzling with olive oil and lemon juice.
4. Top the salad with flaked salmon.

Serving: 1 serving

Nutritional Value: Calories: 250, Protein: 22g, Calcium: 200mg

Cooking Time: 15 minutes

6. Quinoa and Black Bean Bowl

Ingredients:

- ❖ 1/2 cup cooked quinoa
- ❖ 1/2 cup black beans, drained and rinsed
- ❖ 1/4 cup diced red bell pepper
- ❖ 1/4 cup corn kernels
- ❖ 1/4 cup diced avocado
- ❖ 1 tablespoon fresh lime juice
- ❖ 1/2 teaspoon cumin
- ❖ Salt and pepper to taste

Preparation:

1. In a bowl, combine cooked quinoa, black beans, red bell pepper, corn, and avocado.
2. Drizzle with fresh lime juice and sprinkle with cumin.
3. Season with salt and pepper and toss well.

Serving: 1 serving

Nutritional Value: Calories: 300, Protein: 11g, Calcium: 40mg

Cooking Time: 20 minutes (for quinoa preparation)

Ingredients:

- ❖ 1/2 cup dried green or brown lentils
- ❖ 1 cup mixed vegetables (carrots, celery, onions)
- ❖ 1 clove garlic, minced
- ❖ 4 cups low-sodium vegetable broth
- ❖ 1/2 teaspoon thyme
- ❖ Pinch of Salt and pepper to taste

Preparation:

1. Rinse and drain lentils.
2. In a pot, sauté mixed vegetables and garlic until soft.
3. Add lentils, vegetable broth, thyme, and season with salt and pepper.
4. Cook for twenty-five to thirty minutes or until the lentils are cooked.

Serving: 2 servings

Nutritional Value (per serving): Calories: 220, Protein: 10g, Calcium: 40mg

Cooking Time: 45 minutes

8. Grilled Chicken and Asparagus

Ingredients:

- ❖ 4 oz grilled chicken breast
- ❖ 1 cup asparagus spears
- ❖ 1/2 tablespoon olive oil
- ❖ 1/2 teaspoon garlic powder
- ❖ Lemon wedges for garnish
- ❖ Small Salt and pepper to taste

Preparation:

1. Season the chicken breast with garlic powder, salt, and pepper.
2. Grill the chicken until fully cooked.
3. In a separate pan, sauté asparagus in olive oil until tender.
4. Serve the grilled chicken with asparagus and garnish with lemon wedges.

Serving: 1 serving

Nutritional Value: Calories: 280, Protein: 30g, Calcium: 40mg

Cooking Time: 20 minutes

9. Tuna and White Bean Salad

Ingredients:

- ❖ 3 oz canned tuna in water, drained
- ❖ 1/2 cup canned white beans, drained and rinsed
- ❖ 1/4 cup diced red onion
- ❖ 1/4 cup chopped parsley
- ❖ 1 tablespoon olive oil and red wine vinegar
- ❖ Salt and pepper to taste

Preparation:

1. In a bowl, combine canned tuna, white beans, red onion, and parsley.
2. Drizzle with red wine vinegar and olive oil.
3. Season with salt and pepper, and mix to combine.

Serving: 1 serving

Nutritional Value: Calories: 270, Protein: 30g, Calcium: 100mg

Cooking Time: 10 minute

10. Broccoli and Chickpea Stir-Fry

Ingredients:

- ❖ 1 cup broccoli florets
- ❖ 1/2 cup canned chickpeas, drained and rinsed
- ❖ 1/4 cup sliced red bell pepper
- ❖ 1/4 cup sliced mushrooms
- ❖ 2 tablespoons low-sodium soy sauce
- ❖ 1 teaspoon sesame oil
- ❖ 1/2 teaspoon ginger

Preparation:

1. In a pan, stir-fry broccoli, chickpeas, red bell pepper, and mushrooms with sesame oil and ginger until tender.
2. Drizzle with low-sodium soy sauce and stir-fry for an additional minute.

Serving: 1 serving

Nutritional Value: Calories: 280, Protein: 12g, Calcium: 50mg

Cooking Time: 15 minutes

1. Lentil and Spinach Curry

Ingredients:

- ❖ 1/2 cup dried green lentils
- ❖ 1 cup fresh spinach
- ❖ 1/2 cup diced tomatoes
- ❖ 1/4 cup diced onions
- ❖ 1 clove garlic, minced
- ❖ 1 teaspoon curry powder
- ❖ Salt and pepper to taste

Preparation:

1. Rinse and drain lentils.
2. Add the garlic and onions to a saucepan and cook until tender.
3. Add diced tomatoes, curry powder, salt, and pepper.
4. Stir in lentils and simmer for 20-25 minutes until lentils are tender.
5. Add fresh spinach and cook until wilted.

Serving: 2 servings

Nutritional Value (per serving): Calories: 280, Protein: 15g, Calcium: 40mg

Cooking Time: 45 minutes

Ingredients:

- ❖ 4 oz ground turkey
- ❖ 1 cup mixed vegetables (e.g., broccoli, bell peppers, snap peas)
- ❖ 1/4 cup sliced mushrooms
- ❖ 1/4 cup low-sodium teriyaki sauce
- ❖ 1 teaspoon sesame oil, 1/2 teaspoon ginger

Preparation:

1. Cook the ground turkey in a pan until browned.
2. Add mixed vegetables and mushrooms, stir-fry until tender.
3. Drizzle with teriyaki sauce and sesame oil.
4. Sprinkle with ginger and cook for an additional minute.

Serving: 1 serving

Nutritional Value: Calories: 290, Protein: 20g, Calcium: 60mg

Cooking Time: 15 minutes

3. Stuffed Acorn Squash

Ingredients:

- ❖ 1 acorn squash, halved and seeds removed
- ❖ 1/2 cup cooked quinoa
- ❖ 1/4 cup chopped walnuts
- ❖ 1/4 cup dried cranberries
- ❖ 1/2 teaspoon cinnamon
- ❖ Salt and pepper to taste

Preparation:

1. Preheat the oven to 375°F (190°C).
2. The Acorn Squash halves should be put on a baking pan.
3. In a bowl, combine cooked quinoa, chopped walnuts, dried cranberries, cinnamon, salt, and pepper.
4. Stuff the acorn squash halves with the quinoa mixture.
5. Bake the squash for thirty to thirty-five minutes, or until it is soft.

Serving: 2 servings

Nutritional Value (per serving): Calories: 270, Protein: 6g, Calcium: 80mg

Cooking Time: 45 minutes

4. Chicken and Vegetable Skewers

Ingredients:

- ❖ 4 oz chicken breast, cut into chunks
- ❖ 1 cup bell pepper chunks
- ❖ 1/2 cup red onion chunks
- ❖ 1/2 cup zucchini chunks
- ❖ 1 tablespoon olive oil
- ❖ 1/2 teaspoon garlic powder
- ❖ Salt and pepper to taste

Preparation:

1. Preheat the grill or use a grill pan.
2. Thread chicken and vegetables onto skewers.
3. Add a drizzle of olive oil and season with salt, pepper, and garlic powder.
4. Grill for 10-15 minutes, or until chicken is cooked through and vegetables are tender.

Serving: 2 servings

Nutritional Value (per serving): Calories: 260, Protein: 30g, Calcium: 40mg

Cooking Time: 15 minutes

5. Chickpea and Spinach Curry

Ingredients:

- ❖ 1/2 cup canned chickpeas, drained and rinsed
- ❖ 1 cup fresh spinach
- ❖ 1/4 cup diced tomatoes
- ❖ 1/4 cup diced onions
- ❖ 1 clove garlic, minced
- ❖ 1 teaspoon curry powder
- ❖ Salt and pepper to taste

Preparation:

1. Add the garlic and onions to a saucepan and cook until tender.
2. Add diced tomatoes, curry powder, salt, and pepper.
3. Stir in chickpeas and simmer for 10-15 minutes.
4. Add fresh spinach and cook until wilted.

Serving: 2 servings

Nutritional Value (per serving): Calories: 240, Protein:8g, Calcium: 80mg

Cooking Time: 30 minutes

6. Tofu and Vegetable Stir-Fry

Ingredients:

- ❖ 4 oz firm tofu, cubed
- ❖ 1 cup mixed vegetables (e.g., broccoli, carrots, snap peas)
- ❖ 1/4 cup sliced mushrooms
- ❖ 2 tablespoons low-sodium soy sauce
- ❖ 1 teaspoon sesame oil, 1/2 teaspoon ginger

Preparation:

1. In a pan, stir-fry tofu until golden.
2. Add mixed vegetables and mushrooms, stir-fry until tender.
3. Drizzle with sesame oil and low-sodium soy sauce.
4. Sprinkle with ginger and cook for an additional minute.

Serving: 1 serving

Nutritional Value: Calories: 280, Protein: 18g, Calcium: 60mg

Cooking Time: 15 minutes

7. Salmon and Broccoli Foil Pack

Ingredients:

- ❖ 4 oz salmon fillet
- ❖ 1 cup broccoli florets
- ❖ 1/2 cup sliced red bell pepper
- ❖ 1/2 tablespoon olive oil
- ❖ 1/2 teaspoon lemon zest
- ❖ Salt and pepper to taste

Preparation:

1. Preheat the oven to 375°F (190°C).
2. Place salmon, broccoli, and red bell pepper on a large piece of aluminum foil.
3. Drizzle with olive oil, lemon zest, and season with salt and pepper.
4. Seal the foil into a packet and bake for 20-25 minutes, until the salmon is cooked through.

Serving: 1 serving

Nutritional Value: Calories: 290, Protein: 25g, Calcium: 60mg

Cooking Time: 25 minutes

Ingredients:

- ❖ 1/2 cup cooked quinoa
- ❖ 1 cup mixed vegetables (e.g., carrots, celery, green beans)
- ❖ 1/4 cup diced onions
- ❖ 1 clove garlic, minced
- ❖ 4 cups low-sodium vegetable broth
- ❖ 1/2 teaspoon thyme
- ❖ Salt and pepper to taste

Preparation:

1. Add the garlic and onions to a saucepan and cook until tender.
2. Add mixed vegetables, quinoa, vegetable broth, thyme, salt, and pepper.
3. Simmer for 20-25 minutes until vegetables are tender.

Serving: 2 servings

Nutritional Value (per serving): Calories: 230, Protein: 6g, Calcium: 40mg

Cooking Time: 45 minutes

9. Baked Lemon Herb Tilapia

Ingredients:

- ❖ 4 oz tilapia fillet, 1 lemon, thinly sliced
- ❖ 1 teaspoon olive oil
- ❖ 1/2 teaspoon dried herbs (e.g., thyme, rosemary, oregano)
- ❖ Salt and pepper to taste

Preparation:

1. Preheat the oven to 375°F (190°C).
2. Place the tilapia fillet on a baking sheet.
3. Drizzle with olive oil, sprinkle with dried herbs, and season with salt and pepper.
4. Top with lemon slices.
5. Bake the fish for fifteen to twenty minutes, or until it is flaky.

Serving: 1 serving

Nutritional Value: Calories: 220, Protein: 25g, Calcium: 40mg

Cooking Time: 20 minutes

10. Quinoa and Vegetable Stuffed Bell Peppers

Ingredients:

- ❖ 2 large bell peppers
- ❖ 1/2 cup cooked quinoa
- ❖ 1/4 cup black beans, drained and rinsed
- ❖ 1/4 cup diced tomatoes
- ❖ 1/4 cup diced zucchini
- ❖ 1/4 cup low-sodium vegetable broth
- ❖ 1/2 teaspoon cumin
- ❖ Salt and pepper to taste

Preparation:

1. Preheat the oven to 375°F (190°C).
2. Remove the seeds and cut off the bell peppers' tops.
3. In a bowl, combine cooked quinoa, black beans, diced tomatoes, diced zucchini, vegetable broth, cumin, salt, and pepper.
4. Place the quinoa mixture inside the bell peppers.
5. The filled peppers should be put on a baking tray and covered with foil.
6. Bake the peppers for thirty to thirty-five minutes, or until they are soft.

Serving: 2 servings

Nutritional Value (per serving):

Calories: 250

Protein: 8g

Calcium: 60mg

Cooking Time: 45 minutes

1. Apple Cinnamon Spice Smoothie

Ingredients:

- ❖ 1 apple, cored and sliced
- ❖ 1/2 teaspoon ground cinnamon
- ❖ 1/2 cup low-fat Greek yogurt
- ❖ 1/2 cup almond milk (unsweetened)
- ❖ 1 tablespoon oats

Preparation:

1. Blend apple slices, ground cinnamon, low-fat Greek yogurt, almond milk, and oats until smooth.

Serving: 1 serving

Nutritional Value:

Calories: 200

Protein: 8g

Calcium: 220mg

Ingredients:

- ❖ 1/2 cup pomegranate seeds
- ❖ 1/2 cup mixed berries (blueberries, strawberries, raspberries)
- ❖ 1/2 cup low-fat Greek yogurt
- ❖ 1/2 cup water

Preparation:

1. Blend pomegranate seeds, mixed berries, low-fat Greek yogurt, and water until smooth.

Serving: 1 serving

3. Berry Bliss Smoothie

Ingredients:

- ❖ 1/2 cup mixed berries (blueberries, strawberries, raspberries)
- ❖ 1/2 cup low-fat Greek yogurt
- ❖ 1/2 cup almond milk (unsweetened)
- ❖ 1 tablespoon chia seeds
- ❖ 1 teaspoon honey (optional)

Preparation:

1. Blend mixed berries, Greek yogurt, almond milk, and chia seeds until smooth.
2. Add honey for sweetness if desired.

Serving: 1 serving

Nutritional Value:

Calories: 180

Protein: 12g

Calcium: 250mg

4. Green Goddess Smoothie

Ingredients:

- ❖ 1 cup fresh spinach
- ❖ 1/2 cup pineapple chunks
- ❖ 1/2 banana
- ❖ 1/2 cup low-fat Greek yogurt
- ❖ 1/2 cup water

Preparation:

1. Blend fresh spinach, pineapple chunks, banana, low-fat Greek yogurt, and water until smooth.

Serving: 1 serving

Nutritional Value:

Calories: 180

Protein: 10g

Calcium: 220mg

Ingredients:

- ❖ 1 cup fresh kale
- ❖ 2 kiwis, peeled and sliced
- ❖ 1/2 cup low-fat Greek yogurt
- ❖ 1/2 cup water

Preparation:

1. Blend fresh kale, kiwis, low-fat Greek yogurt, and water until smooth.

Serving: 1 serving

Nutritional Value:

Calories: 190

Protein: 9g

Calcium: 200mg

6. Berry Banana Boost Smoothie

Ingredients:

- ❖ 1/2 cup mixed berries (blueberries, strawberries, raspberries)
- ❖ 1/2 banana
- ❖ 1/2 cup low-fat Greek yogurt
- ❖ 1/2 cup almond milk (unsweetened)
- ❖ 1 tablespoon flaxseeds

Preparation:

1. Blend mixed berries, banana, low-fat Greek yogurt, almond milk, and flaxseeds until smooth.

Serving: 1 serving

Nutritional Value:

Calories: 190

Protein: 12g

Calcium: 230mg

Ingredients:

- ❖ 2 large carrots
- ❖ 1-inch piece of fresh ginger
- ❖ 1 apple, cored and sliced
- ❖ 1/2 lemon, peeled

Preparation:

1. Juice the carrots, ginger, apple, and lemon.
2. Stir well and serve over ice.

Serving: 1 serving

Nutritional Value:

Calories: 120

Protein: 2g

Calcium: 60mg

8. Creamy Avocado Green Smoothie

Ingredients:

- ❖ 1/2 avocado
- ❖ 1 cup fresh spinach
- ❖ 1/2 banana
- ❖ 1/2 cup almond milk (unsweetened)
- ❖ 1/2 cup low-fat Greek yogurt
- ❖ 1 teaspoon honey (optional)

Preparation:

1. Blend avocado, fresh spinach, banana, almond milk, low-fat Greek yogurt, and honey (if desired) until smooth.

Serving: 1 serving

Nutritional Value:

Calories: 220

Protein: 10g

Calcium: 240mg

Ingredients:

- ❖ 1 orange, peeled
- ❖ 1/2 grapefruit, peeled
- ❖ 1 lemon, peeled
- ❖ 1/2 lime, peeled

Preparation:

1. Juice the orange, grapefruit, lemon, and lime.
2. Stir well and serve over ice.

Serving: 1 serving

Nutritional Value:

Calories: 100

Protein: 2g

Calcium: 60mg

10. Tropical Twist Smoothie

Ingredients:

- ❖ 1/2 cup pineapple chunks
- ❖ 1/2 banana
- ❖ 1/2 cup low-fat coconut milk
- ❖ 1/2 cup low-fat Greek yogurt
- ❖ 1/2 cup water

Preparation:

1. Blend pineapple chunks, banana, low-fat coconut milk, low-fat Greek yogurt, and water until smooth.

Serving: 1 serving

Nutritional Value:

Calories: 200

Protein: 8g

Calcium: 180mg

Not only are these smoothie and juice recipes for seniors delicious, but they are also nutrient-dense, supporting bone health and general well-being. Include them in your daily routine to take advantage of nutrients that have been scientifically established to be effective in controlling osteoporosis. Savor these cool drinks as a tasty complement to your osteoporosis diet.

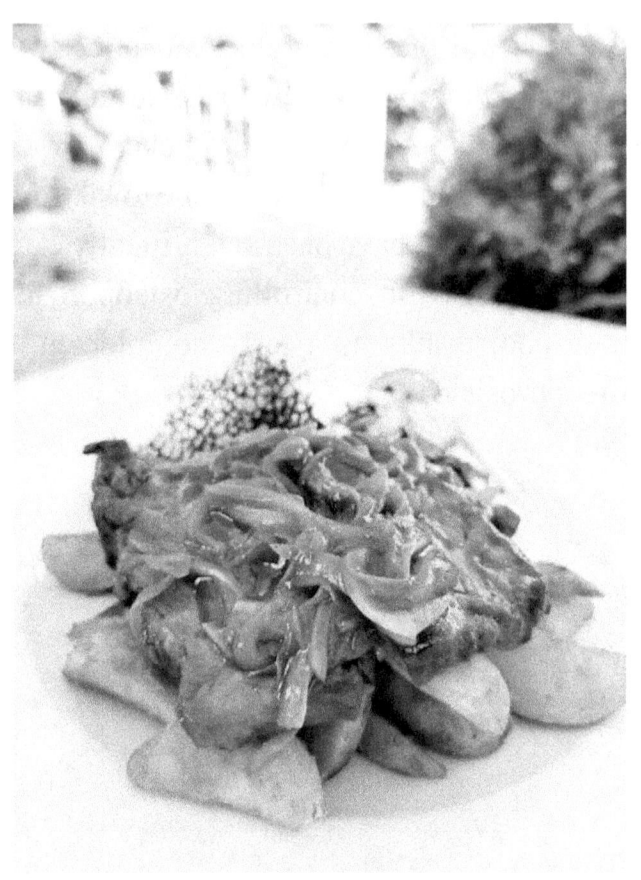

CONCLUSION

A labor of love, " Osteoporosis Diet Cookbook for Seniors" is painstakingly written to provide you with the information and recipes you need to take control of your overall health and bone health. Although osteoporosis may appear to be an overwhelming enemy, you may overcome it with the correct resources and advice.

We have discussed the nature of osteoporosis, its causes, symptoms, and preventive methods throughout this cookbook. We've discussed the significance of eating a tasty, scientifically-proven diet to control osteoporosis. You've stumbled across a veritable gold mine of nutrient-dense meals, ranging from breakfast to dinner, juice to smoothies, all thoughtfully crafted to bolster bone health and complement kidney- and diabetes-friendly, heart-healthy diets. This is about adopting a lifestyle that enables you to live life to the fullest, not just about sticking to a diet. It's about enjoying each taste of these delectable recipes with the knowledge that each one is a step toward better health, stronger bones, and a more rewarding future.

Picture yourself as more confident, more nimble, and ready to take on life's adventures.

Imagine yourself enjoying the mouthwatering tastes of these recipes and knowing that each bite is nourishing your body and preventing osteoporosis.

This cookbook is your reliable guide, and you are the master of your own health. Accept it, try out the recipes, and incorporate them into your everyday life. The decision you made today will be appreciated by your bones and by your future self.

Don't wait, my dear reader. Set out on this path to healthier bones and a livelier existence. You hold the power, and I have faith that you can succeed. You are powerful, and every recipe you make from these pages is the first step on your path to a happier, healthier life.

.

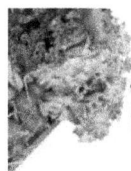

WEEKLY MEAL PLANNER

			GROCERY LIST
MONDAY	BREAKFAST		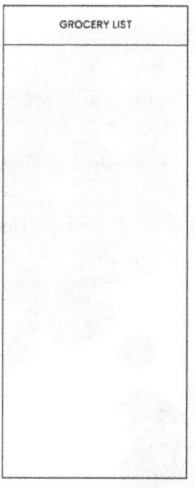
	LUNCH		
	DINNER		
TUESDAY	BREAKFAST		
	LUNCH		
	DINNER		
WEDNESDAY	BREAKFAST		
	LUNCH		
	DINNER		
THURSDAY	BREAKFAST		
	LUNCH		
	DINNER		
FRIDAY	BREAKFAST		SNACKS
	LUNCH		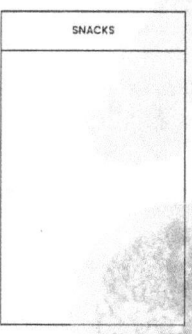
	DINNER		
SARTURDAY	BREAKFAST		
	LUNCH		
	DINNER		
SUNDAY	BREAKFAST		
	LUNCH		
	DINNER		

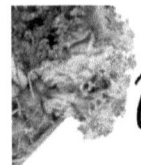

WEEKLY MEAL PLANNER

			GROCERY LIST
MONDAY	BREAKFAST		
	LUNCH		
	DINNER		
TUESDAY	BREAKFAST		
	LUNCH		
	DINNER		
WEDNESDAY	BREAKFAST		
	LUNCH		
	DINNER		
THURSDAY	BREAKFAST		
	LUNCH		
	DINNER		
FRIDAY	BREAKFAST		SNACKS
	LUNCH		
	DINNER		
SARTURDAY	BREAKFAST		
	LUNCH		
	DINNER		
SUNDAY	BREAKFAST		
	LUNCH		
	DINNER		

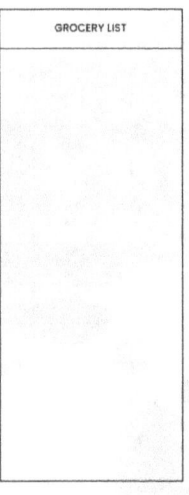

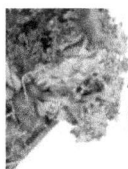

WEEKLY MEAL PLANNER

MONDAY	BREAKFAST	
	LUNCH	
	DINNER	
TUESDAY	BREAKFAST	
	LUNCH	
	DINNER	
WEDNESDAY	BREAKFAST	
	LUNCH	
	DINNER	
THURSDAY	BREAKFAST	
	LUNCH	
	DINNER	
FRIDAY	BREAKFAST	
	LUNCH	
	DINNER	
SARTURDAY	BREAKFAST	
	LUNCH	
	DINNER	
SUNDAY	BREAKFAST	
	LUNCH	
	DINNER	

GROCERY LIST

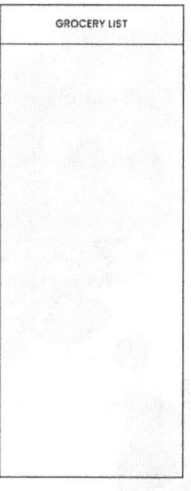

SNACKS

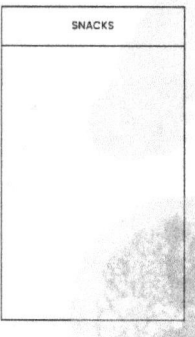

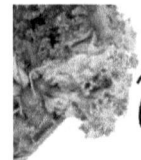

WEEKLY MEAL PLANNER

				GROCERY LIST
MONDAY	BREAKFAST			
	LUNCH			
	DINNER			
TUESDAY	BREAKFAST			
	LUNCH			
	DINNER			
WEDNESDAY	BREAKFAST			
	LUNCH			
	DINNER			
THURSDAY	BREAKFAST			
	LUNCH			
	DINNER			
FRIDAY	BREAKFAST			
	LUNCH			
	DINNER			
SARTURDAY	BREAKFAST			
	LUNCH			
	DINNER			
SUNDAY	BREAKFAST			
	LUNCH			
	DINNER			

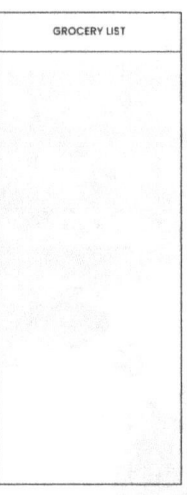

GROCERY LIST

SNACKS

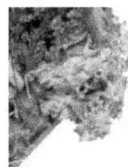

WEEKLY MEAL PLANNER

			GROCERY LIST
MONDAY	BREAKFAST		
	LUNCH		
	DINNER		
TUESDAY	BREAKFAST		
	LUNCH		
	DINNER		
WEDNESDAY	BREAKFAST		
	LUNCH		
	DINNER		
THURSDAY	BREAKFAST		
	LUNCH		
	DINNER		
FRIDAY	BREAKFAST		
	LUNCH		SNACKS
	DINNER		
SARTURDAY	BREAKFAST		
	LUNCH		
	DINNER		
SUNDAY	BREAKFAST		
	LUNCH		
	DINNER		

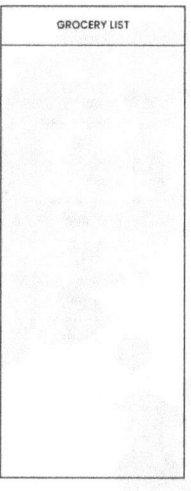

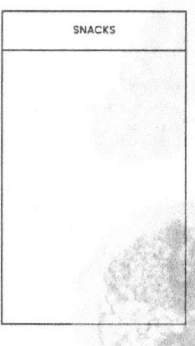

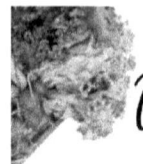

WEEKY MEAl PlANNER

			GROCERY LIST
MONDAY	BREAKFAST		
	LUNCH		
	DINNER		
TUESDAY	BREAKFAST		
	LUNCH		
	DINNER		
WEDNESDAY	BREAKFAST		
	LUNCH		
	DINNER		
THURSDAY	BREAKFAST		
	LUNCH		
	DINNER		
FRIDAY	BREAKFAST		
	LUNCH		
	DINNER		
SARTURDAY	BREAKFAST		
	LUNCH		
	DINNER		
SUNDAY	BREAKFAST		
	LUNCH		
	DINNER		

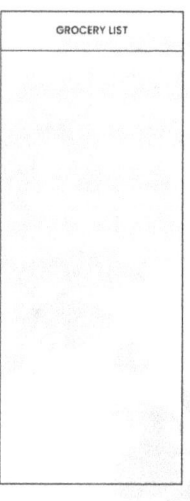

SNACKS

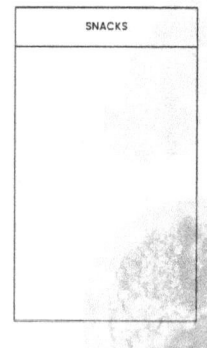

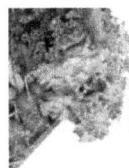

WEEKLY MEAL PLANNER

				GROCERY LIST
MONDAY	BREAKFAST			
	LUNCH			
	DINNER			
TUESDAY	BREAKFAST			
	LUNCH			
	DINNER			
WEDNESDAY	BREAKFAST			
	LUNCH			
	DINNER			
THURSDAY	BREAKFAST			
	LUNCH			
	DINNER			
FRIDAY	BREAKFAST			
	LUNCH			SNACKS
	DINNER			
SARTURDAY	BREAKFAST			
	LUNCH			
	DINNER			
SUNDAY	BREAKFAST			
	LUNCH			
	DINNER			

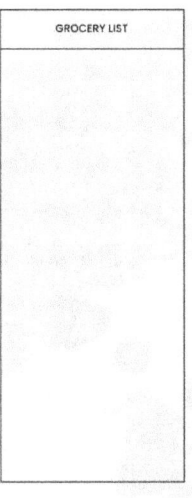

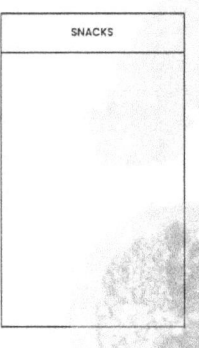

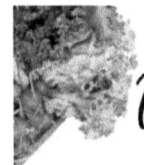

WEEKLY MEAL PLANNER

			GROCERY LIST
MONDAY	BREAKFAST		
	LUNCH		
	DINNER		
TUESDAY	BREAKFAST		
	LUNCH		
	DINNER		
WEDNESDAY	BREAKFAST		
	LUNCH		
	DINNER		
THURSDAY	BREAKFAST		
	LUNCH		
	DINNER		
FRIDAY	BREAKFAST		SNACKS
	LUNCH		
	DINNER		
SARTURDAY	BREAKFAST		
	LUNCH		
	DINNER		
SUNDAY	BREAKFAST		
	LUNCH		
	DINNER		

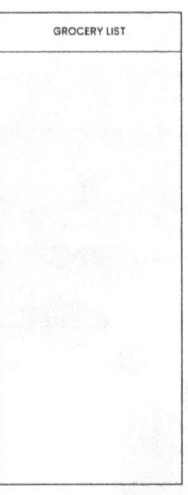

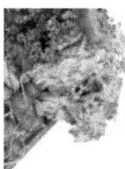

WEEKLY MEAL PLANNER

				GROCERY LIST
MONDAY	BREAKFAST			
	LUNCH			
	DINNER			
TUESDAY	BREAKFAST			
	LUNCH			
	DINNER			
WEDNESDAY	BREAKFAST			
	LUNCH			
	DINNER			
THURSDAY	BREAKFAST			
	LUNCH			
	DINNER			
FRIDAY	BREAKFAST			
	LUNCH			SNACKS
	DINNER			
SARTURDAY	BREAKFAST			
	LUNCH			
	DINNER			
SUNDAY	BREAKFAST			
	LUNCH			
	DINNER			

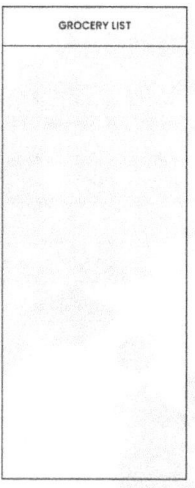

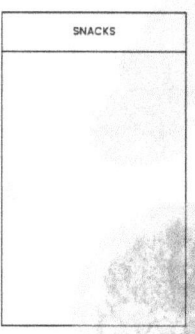

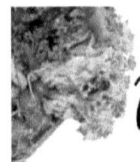

WEEKLY MEAL PLANNER

			GROCERY LIST
MONDAY	BREAKFAST		
	LUNCH		
	DINNER		
TUESDAY	BREAKFAST		
	LUNCH		
	DINNER		
WEDNESDAY	BREAKFAST		
	LUNCH		
	DINNER		
THURSDAY	BREAKFAST		
	LUNCH		
	DINNER		
FRIDAY	BREAKFAST		SNACKS
	LUNCH		
	DINNER		
SARTURDAY	BREAKFAST		
	LUNCH		
	DINNER		
SUNDAY	BREAKFAST		
	LUNCH		
	DINNER		

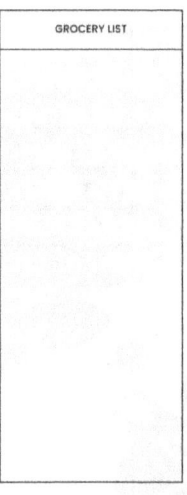

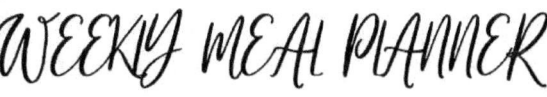

WEEKLY MEAL PLANNER

MONDAY	BREAKFAST	
	LUNCH	
	DINNER	
TUESDAY	BREAKFAST	
	LUNCH	
	DINNER	
WEDNESDAY	BREAKFAST	
	LUNCH	
	DINNER	
THURSDAY	BREAKFAST	
	LUNCH	
	DINNER	
FRIDAY	BREAKFAST	
	LUNCH	
	DINNER	
SARTURDAY	BREAKFAST	
	LUNCH	
	DINNER	
SUNDAY	BREAKFAST	
	LUNCH	
	DINNER	

GROCERY LIST

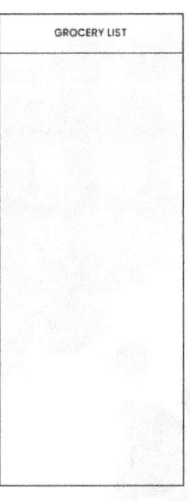

SNACKS

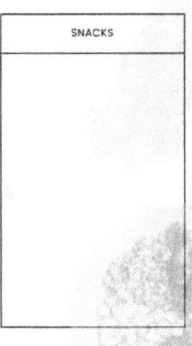

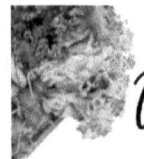

WEEKLY MEAL PLANNER

MONDAY	BREAKFAST		
	LUNCH		
	DINNER		
TUESDAY	BREAKFAST		
	LUNCH		
	DINNER		
WEDNESDAY	BREAKFAST		
	LUNCH		
	DINNER		
THURSDAY	BREAKFAST		
	LUNCH		
	DINNER		
FRIDAY	BREAKFAST		
	LUNCH		
	DINNER		
SARTURDAY	BREAKFAST		
	LUNCH		
	DINNER		
SUNDAY	BREAKFAST		
	LUNCH		
	DINNER		

GROCERY LIST

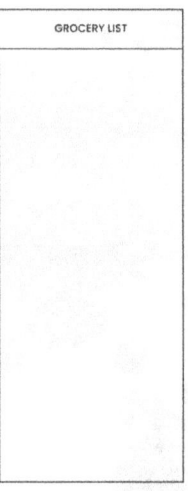

SNACKS

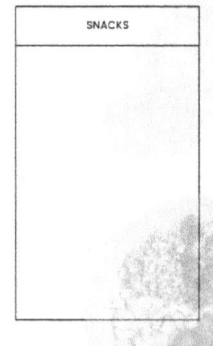

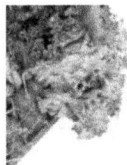

WEEKLY MEAL PLANNER

			GROCERY LIST
MONDAY	BREAKFAST		
	LUNCH		
	DINNER		
TUESDAY	BREAKFAST		
	LUNCH		
	DINNER		
WEDNESDAY	BREAKFAST		
	LUNCH		
	DINNER		
THURSDAY	BREAKFAST		
	LUNCH		
	DINNER		
FRIDAY	BREAKFAST		
	LUNCH		SNACKS
	DINNER		
SARTURDAY	BREAKFAST		
	LUNCH		
	DINNER		
SUNDAY	BREAKFAST		
	LUNCH		
	DINNER		

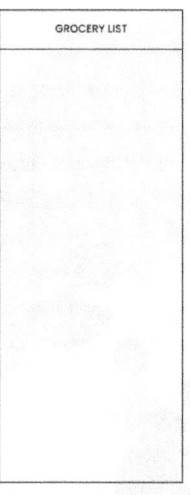

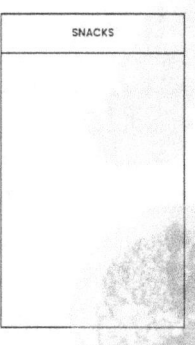

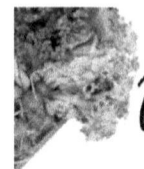

WEEKLY MEAL PLANNER

			GROCERY LIST
MONDAY	BREAKFAST		
	LUNCH		
	DINNER		
TUESDAY	BREAKFAST		
	LUNCH		
	DINNER		
WEDNESDAY	BREAKFAST		
	LUNCH		
	DINNER		
THURSDAY	BREAKFAST		
	LUNCH		
	DINNER		
FRIDAY	BREAKFAST		
	LUNCH		
	DINNER		
SARTURDAY	BREAKFAST		
	LUNCH		
	DINNER		
SUNDAY	BREAKFAST		
	LUNCH		
	DINNER		

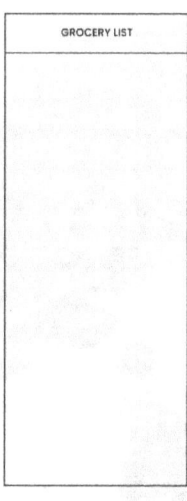

SNACKS

www.ingramcontent.com/pod-product-compliance
Lightning Source LLC
Chambersburg PA
CBHW070434290526
45791CB00005B/1970